Spiralize

100% VEGAN

Energizing Spiralizer Recipes for Weight Loss, Detox, and Optimal Health

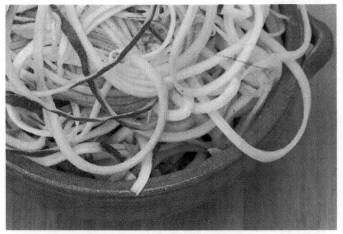

By Karen Greenvang
Copyright ©Karen Greenvang 2016

Free Vegan eBook Available at:
www.HolisticWellnessBooks.com/vegan

otherwise, without the prior written permission of the author and the publishers.

other qualified health professionals regarding the treatment of medical conditions. The author shall not be held liable or responsible for any misunderstanding or misuse of the information contained in this book. The information is not intended to diagnose, treat or cure any disease.

It is important to remember that the author of this book is not a doctor/ medical professional. Only opinions based upon her own personal experiences or research are cited. THE AUTHOR DOES NOT OFFER MEDICAL ADVICE or prescribe any treatments. For any health or medical issues – you should be talking to your doctor first.

Table of Contents

Introduction

1951's Vegan Society definition of veganism: "Veganism is the doctrine that humans should live without exploiting animals."

Vegan cuisine is based on the exclusion of all animal products, including meat, eggs, dairy, honey, gelatin etc. Many people are aware of the abuse inflicted on animals and would like to experiment with a healthier diet, that is environmentally conscious and cautious and respectful of animals. Often people are discouraged by the lack of recipes or tools to achieve it. This book attempts to address this problem and also to supplement the needs of long-time vegans who would like to add a variety of textures and looks to their dishes.

The use of the spiralizer gives any dish an interesting twist and changes textures and possibilities of any meal. The spiralizer is an essential to the raw food kitchen, as it takes its place in our kitchens, it will keep for a long time as an important kitchen utensil. For children, eating vegetables will become tastier and more amusing. From the age of seven years, they can use the device and participate in the preparation of the meals.

If you wish to eat less pasta because of the calorie or gluten content, vegetables can take its place advantageously without missing out on your favorite recipes. The spiralizer in vegan cooking is a perfect edition to your meal plan.

A lot of vegetables and some fruits can be spiralized, such as:

- Beets,
- apples,
- carrots,
- celeriac,
- turnips,
- parsnips,
- radish,
- cucumber,
- rutabaga,
- daikon radish,
- persimmons,
- jicama,
- onions,
- chayote,
- potatoes,
- kohlrabi,

- dragon fruit,
- broccoli,
- zucchini,
- cabbage,
- eddoes,
- butternut squash,
- sweet potatoes,
- plantains and even pears.

You can also try Jerusalem Artichoke, or yam and cassava although the last two must be cooked after for the starch they contain and might break their spirals a bit.

Raw, boiled, steamed or sautéed, spiralized veggies are a great accompaniment to any meal and add great flavor. The spiralizer is a must have device in any vegan (and even non-vegan) kitchen!

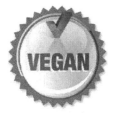 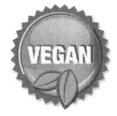

Free Complimentary eBook

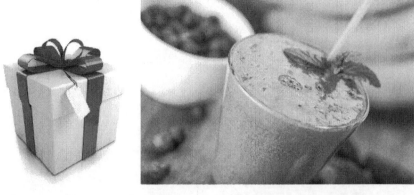

Before we dive into the recipes, I would like to offer you a free, complimentary recipe eBook with delicious vegan superfood smoothies.

Download it now, before you forget:

www.holisticwellnessbooks.com/vegan

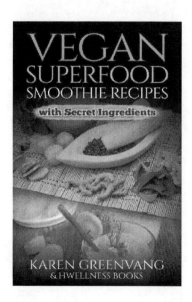

If you have any problems with your download, email me at:
karenveganbooks@gmail.com

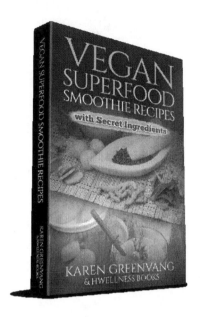

www.holisticwellnessbooks.com/vegan

Recipe Measurements

I love keeping ingredient measurements as simple as possible-this is why in many of my recipes, I stick to tablespoons, teaspoons and cups.

If you don't have American Cup measures, just use a metric or imperial liquid measuring jug and fill your jug with your ingredient to the corresponding level. Here's how to go about it:

1 American Cup= 250ml= 8 fl.oz

Pounds to grams (lb. to g.): 1 lb= 450g.

Translations

Eggplant=Aubergine

Zucchini=Courgette

Cilantro=Coriander

Garbanzo Beans=Chickpeas

Navy Beans-=Haricot Beans

Aragula=Rocket

Broth=Stock

Your Unique Recipes

Breakfast

Sweet Vegan Potato Scones on a Bed of Spiralized Apples

<u>Serves: 2</u>

<u>Ingredients:</u>

- ½ lb. boiled and mashed potatoes
- 1 oz. plain or all-purpose flour
- 1 oz. almond or soy butter (I prefer almond)
- ½ tsp salt
- Pinch of pepper
- ½ tsp of baking powder
- A pinch of cinnamon
- ½ cup of maple syrup
- 2 spiralized apples to serve

Preparation:

1. In a medium pan, add water to fill half of the pan and add salt and the potatoes. Boil until soft.
2. Drain the potatoes and mash them with the soy or almond butter, salt, pepper, cinnamon and baking powder.
3. Make a firm dough, by mixing in the flour to the mixture. Add more if the dough is too sloppy.
4. On a floured board roll out the dough to a thickness of 5mm.
5. Using a coffee plate cut out as many rounds as the dough will stretch to.
6. Score the dough to mark 4 equal wedges and also prick all over with a fork.
7. Lightly grease a wok and fry the dough.
8. Fry each side for a few minutes on a medium heat so that they are golden brown and crispy.
9. Sprinkle with maple syrup and serve on a bed of spiralized apples.

Chia, Coconut and Blueberry Pudding with a Spiralized Pear Topping

Serves: 1-2

Ingredients:

- 2 tbsp. chia seeds
- 1 tbsp. coconut milk powder
- 1 tbsp. maple syrup

Toppings:

- Half a cup of blueberries
- 1 pear spiralized

Preparation:

1. Grind the chia seeds in a blender with a grinder attachment like if you wanted to grind coffee beans.
2. Add the coconut milk powder and water and heat to boiling point. You can omit this step if you want it to be a cold pudding.
3. Whisk the ground chia seeds into the liquid. Whisk again after a few minutes. Leave the mixture until it thickens and serve with a drizzle of maple syrup. Top it with blueberries and a spiralized pear for a delicious breakfast or in-between meals during the day.

Spiralized Celery Root, Parsnip and Sweet Potato Rosti

<u>Serves: 2</u>

<u>Ingredients:</u>

- 1 cup all-purpose flour
- 1 cup club soda
- ½ oz. silken tofu
- Salt and pepper
- cup finely spiralized celery root
- 1 cup of finely spiralized parsnip
- 2 cups finely spiralized sweet potato
- Oil for cooking

<u>Preparation:</u>

1. Puree the flour, club soda and silken tofu (use a food processor or a blender) until smooth. Lightly season and place to one side.

2. Add the spiralized celery root, sweet potato and parsnip to the batter and stir well to coat. Heat a sauté pan over medium high heat and grease lightly.

3. Add a layer of the rosti mix onto the pan.

4. Bake for a few minutes and take out to apply the next layer. Repeat until the batter is used up. Serve hot.

Budwig Cream

Ingredients:

- 1 ripe banana
- 2 tbsp. freshly ground flaxseeds
- 2 tbsp. fresh whole-wheat rice, millet, buckwheat, oats
- 1 tbsp. of lemon juice
- 1 tbsp. of chia seeds
- 2 tbsp. of almond milk

Preparation:

1. Grind the seeds and nuts (use a coffee grinder). Mash the bananas with a fork and add the ground seeds and lemon juice.
2. Mix well and add a little almond milk as you go. According to your taste, you can add a little maple syrup, a few drops of linseed oil (=flaxseed oil), spiralized fresh fruit or other toppings.

Lunch Recipes

Raw Thai Salad with Spiralized Zucchini

Serves: 2

Ingredients:

- 2 medium zucchini, noodles
- 2 carrots, noodle
- ½ cup green onions (shallots), finely chopped
- 1 medium bell pepper, julienned
- 1 cup finely chopped red cabbage
- 1 green apple julienned
- 1 cup of cauliflower cut into small pieces

Put everything in a large bowl.

Sauce:

- 4 dates soaked in warm water for about thirty minutes (you can substitute dried tomatoes)
- ½ cup butter nuts (almonds, cashews, or even peanuts)
- 3 tbsp. of agave nectar
- 3 tbsp. tamari (soy sauce)
- Juice of one lime

- 1 tsp chili pepper or chili sauce to taste. Garnish with spiralized zucchini.

Preparation:

1. Place ingredients in a food processor and blend until it sounds sauce. If too thick, add a little water.
2. Pour over vegetables. Mix well.
3. Garnish with tomato wedges, coriander, sesame seeds and sunflower seeds. Serve and wait for marriage proposals, lol.

Beet Salad with a Coconut Dressing

Serves: 2

Ingredients:

•1 cup young coconut water

•5 plum tomatoes, sliced

•1 cup macadamia nuts

•2 beets spiralized on thin setting (regular or golden)

•5 rosemary leaves

Preparation:

1. In a blender blitz the macadamia nuts and coconut water until smooth.

2. Add the spiralized beets on top and garnish with rosemary and sliced plum tomatoes.

Quinoa Salad with Grilled Red Peppers and Spiralized Vegetables

Serves: 2

Ingredients:

Basil and Green Onion Vinaigrette:

- ½ tbsp. of olive oil
- ¼ tbsp. of lemon juice
- 2 cloves of garlic, chopped finely
- ¼ tbsp. of chopped green onions
- ¼ tbsp. of fresh basil, chopped finely
- Salt and black pepper to taste

Quinoa Salad:

- 1 cup. of water
- 1 cup of quinoa
- 1 tbsp. of olive oil
- 5 mushrooms, sliced
- 1 jar of grilled red peppers, cut in strips
- 1 red onion and a carrot cut to the spiralizer
- ¼ cup of black olives, sliced

Preparation:

For the Vinaigrette:

1. In a container, put the olive oil, lemon juice, garlic, green

onions and basil.

2. Close the lid and shake. Then season.

Preparation of the salad:

1. Add water to a medium pan and wait until it begins to boil. Add the quinoa and cook for 10 mins.

2. Drain the quinoa and set aside.

3. In a frying pan, heat the oil.

4. Add mushrooms and cook for 3 minutes or until they are soft.

5. In a salad bowl, mix the quinoa, mushrooms, peppers and onions and carrot in spirals.

6. Add the vinaigrette and mix delicately to coat the ingredients.

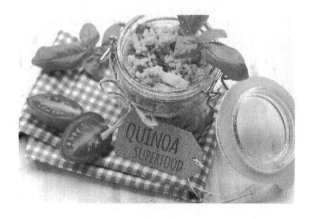

Miso Soup

Serves: 2

Ingredients:

- 4 cups vegetable broth (vegan)
- 3 cups water
- 5 carrots (spiralized)
- ½ head napa cabbage (spiralized, about 2 cups)
- 2 cloves minced garlic
- ½ tsp minced ginger
- 1 tbsp. white miso
- ¼ tsp salt
- 1 handful of greens (a blend of kale and spinach for example)
- 1 zucchini (for later - spiralized)

Preparation:

1. Add carrots, water, broth, cabbage, ginger and garlic to a big saucepan.
2. Stir to combine. Heat up to a boil and then lower the heat to medium-low for about 30 minutes.
3. Once vegetables are cooked, add the greens and zucchini.

4. Let it cook for an additional 5 minutes. Add miso at the last minute to preserve nutrients, then remove from heat and serve.

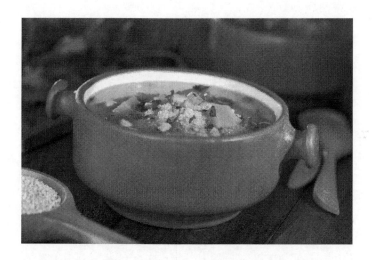

Spiralized Carrot and Cucumber Roast

Ingredients:

- 5 cucumbers, small or medium, peeled, cut lengthwise into 2
- 6 carrots, peeled, spiralized
- 2 tbsp. extra virgin olive oil
- 1 head garlic, cloves in defeat, peeled
- To taste sea salt and freshly ground pepper

Preparation:

1. In a shallow baking dish, pour the oil to coat the bottom. Add the garlic and also season with sea salt and pepper. Add in the vegetables and coat well by stirring in the seasoned oil. Vegetables should be placed in a single layer and not stacked so that they are well roasted. Pour a little olive oil over the vegetables.

2. Preheat the oven to 400 °F (200 Celsius) and cook the vegetables for 15 minutes. Vegetables should be tender and golden.

Root Salad with a Lychee Dressing

Serves: 2

Ingredients:

•1 cup lychee water

•1 cup almond nuts

•2 beetroots spiralized on a regular setting

•5 cherry tomatoes diced

Preparation:

1. Blend lychee water and almond nuts in a blender until smooth.

2. Then, pour it over the veggies.

3. Garnish with chopped tomatoes.

Buckwheat Salad with Spiralized Vegetables

<u>Serves: 2</u>

<u>Ingredients:</u>

<u>Parsley & Green Onion Vinaigrette:</u>

- ½ tbsp. of olive oil
- ¼ tbsp. of balsamic vinegar
- 2 cloves of garlic, chopped finely
- ¼ tbsp. of chopped green onions
- ¼ tbsp. of fresh basil, chopped finely
- Salt and black pepper to taste

<u>Buckwheat Salad:</u>

- 1 cup. of water
- 1 cup of buckwheat
- 1 tbsp. of olive oil
- 5 mushrooms, sliced
- 1 red onion and a carrot, spiralized

<u>Preparation:</u>

<u>For the Vinaigrette:</u>

1. In a container, put the olive oil, balsamic vinegar, garlic, green onions and basil.

2. Close the lid and shake. Then season.

Preparation of the salad:

1. Add water to a medium pan and wait until it begins to boil. Add the buckwheat and cook for 10 mins.

2. Drain the buckwheat and set aside.

3. In a frying pan, heat the oil.

4. Add mushrooms and cook for 3 minutes or until they are soft.

5. In a salad bowl, mix the buckwheat, mushrooms and onions and carrot in spirals.

6. Add the vinaigrette and mix delicately to coat the ingredients. Optional- you could also add some cooked quinoa for more nutrition.

Leek and Mushroom Soup

<u>Serves:</u> 2

<u>Ingredients:</u>

- 1 tbsp. olive oil
- 2 leeks, chopped
- 2 cloves garlic, minced
- 1 ½ lb. mushrooms (nearly 3 cups)
- 1 qt. low-sodium vegetable broth (4 cups)
- ¼ cup chopped cilantro

<u>Carrots and parsnip topping:</u>

- 1 cup of spiralized parsnips, blanched for 2 minutes
- 2 spiralized carrots

<u>Preparation:</u>

1. Heat oil in large saucepan over a medium heat. Add leeks and garlic and sauté for 5 to 7 minutes or until the leeks are soft. Add mushrooms and cook 5 minutes or until most of the liquid has evaporated.
2. Add the vegetable broth, cilantro and simmer for 5 minutes. Reduce heat to medium-low and simmer for 15 more minutes.
3. Purée the soup in batches until smooth.

4. Garnish the soup with spiralized blanched parsnips and carrots.

Ginger and Almond Soup

This soup requires no cooking and can be eaten hot or cold. Adding very thinly spiralized radishes will add a zing to this delicious raw soup.

Ingredients:

- A small piece of fresh ginger
- ½ clove of garlic, peeled and chopped
- Handful of almonds, crushed
- 4 cups of hot water
- A small piece of fresh turmeric
- Handful of fresh parsley
- 3 spiralized radishes

Preparation:

1. Place all the ingredients in a blender and well mix until you obtain a smooth mixture.
2. If you want a hot soup, use hot water instead. Garnish with spiralized radishes.

Spiralized Turnip Soup

Ingredients:

- ½ cup quinoa, soaked
- ½ cup onion, chopped
- 2 red potatoes, spiralized
- 2 turnips, spiralized
- 2 cups kidney beans
- 1 tbsp. of mustard seeds

Preparation:

1. In a medium pan add the soaked quinoa, then cover and bring back to a boil. Lower the heat and simmer for 30 minutes.
2. Add the onion, turnips and potatoes and bring back to a boil, while covered. Lower the heat and simmer for 10 minutes or until all the veggies are tender.
3. Add the kidney beans and mustard seeds and heat until warmed through. Season to taste.

Spicy Pepper Salad

Serves: 1-2

Ingredients:

For the dressing:

•2 yellow and red bell peppers, diced

•1 tbsp. chili powder

•A pinch of paprika powder

•3 tbsp. lime juice

•Sea salt to taste

For the salad:

•3 cups spinach leaves

•1 red bell pepper, spiralized

Preparation:

1. Combine all the ingredients in a high speed blender and blitz until smooth.

2. Place the greens in a salad bowl then scatter the peppers.

3. Lastly, liberally drizzle on the dressing and serve.

Indian Spiralized Celery Salad

Serves: 1-2

Ingredients:

•2 tbsp. of lemon juice

•3 tbsp. coconut cream

•½ tbsp. of vegan mustard

•1 pinch of salt

•1 pinch of ground masala

•½ cup of spiralized celery root (celeriac)

•1 red spiralized apple

Preparation:

1. In a big bowl, lemon juice, mustard and coconut cream until smooth.

2. Add the celery and the apple and mix well until the ingredients are well combined.

Swedish Mushroom Soup

Serves: 1-2

Ingredients:

- 1 tbsp. olive oil
- 2 leeks, chopped
- 2 cloves garlic, minced
- 1 ½ lb. mushrooms
- 1 qt. low-sodium vegetable broth
- 3 fresh thyme strings
- ¼ cup chopped cilantro

Carrots and parsnip topping:

- 1 cup of spiralized carrots and parsnips, blanched for 2 minutes

Preparation:

1. Heat oil in large saucepan over a medium heat. Add leeks and garlic and sauté for 5 to 7 minutes or until the leeks are soft. Add mushrooms and cook 5 minutes or until most of the liquid has evaporated.
2. Add the broth, thyme, cilantro and simmer. Reduce the heat to medium-low and simmer for a further 15 minutes.

3. Purée the soup in batches until smooth and season to your taste.
4. Garnish the soup with spiralized blanched carrots and parsnips.

Raw Carrot, Cashew and Ginger Soup

This soup is easy and fast to realize, it requires no cooking and can be taken hot or cold. It is delicious, smells great, is rich in vitamins and of carotenoids. Adding very thinly spiralized veggies (parsnips, carrots, radish or your choice) will add a zip to this tasteful raw soup.

Serves: 1-2

Ingredients:

- 3 carrots, washed and sliced
- ½ clove of garlic, peeled and chopped
- Handful of cashew nuts
- 250 ml of hot water (more or less 1 cup)
- A small piece of fresh turmeric
- A small piece of fresh ginger
- Handful of fresh coriander

Preparation:

1. Place all the ingredients in a blender and well mix until the obtaining of a smooth and smooth soup.
2. If you want a hot soup, warm your bowl in the bain-marie and opt for some very hot water. Think of realizing your soup at the last minute to benefit all the vitamins and minerals. Sparkle the spiralized veggies of your choice for a maximum boost. C

3. If you want a refreshing gazpacho, place your soup in the refrigerator before serving. For a change, add the juice of one orange or a little bit of oil of almond or hazelnut.

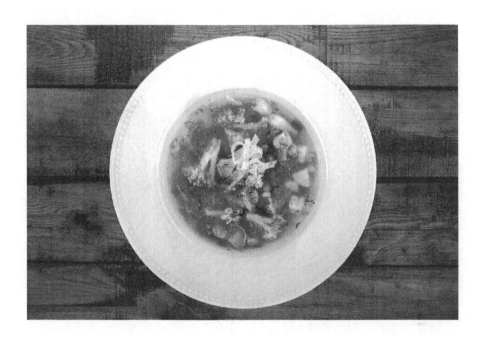

Spiralized Veggie Soup

<u>Serves: 1-2</u>

<u>Ingredients:</u>

- 1/3 cup pre-soaked barley
- ½ cup quinoa, soaked
- ½ cup onion, chopped
- 4 medium carrots, spiralized
- 4 red potatoes, skins on, spiralized
- 2 turnips, spiralized
- 2 cups cooked black beans
- Pinch of celery seeds

<u>Preparation:</u>

1. Place the veggie broth in a large pot and bring to a boil. Add the pre-soaked barley and soaked quinoa, then cover and bring back to a boil. Lower the heat and simmer for 30 minutes.
2. Add the onion, carrots, turnip and potatoes and bring back to a boil, while covered. Lower the heat and simmer for 10 minutes or until all the veggies are tender.
3. Add the cooked black beans and celery seeds and heat until warmed through. Season to taste.

Persimmons Salad

A beautiful winter salad that is rich in phytonutrients and beta carotene from the sweet persimmons.

Serves: 2

Ingredients:

For the dressing:

- 1 yellow or red bell pepper, diced
- 1 ripe persimmon, diced
- 1 tbsp. chili powder
- A pinch of chipotle powder
- 3 tbsp. lime juice
- Sea salt to taste

For the salad:

- 4 cups mixed leaves such as arugula and spinach
- 1 red bell pepper, thinly sliced
- 2 persimmons, sliced

Preparation:

For the dressing:

1. Combine all the ingredients in a blender. Blend well until super smooth.

2. Place the greens in a salad bowl then scatter the red bell

peppers and persimmons.

3. Drizzle on the dressing and serve!

Remember to get your free, complimentary smoothie recipe PDF eBook (100% vegan):

www.holisticwellnessbooks.com/vegan

Fennel and Apple Salad

Serves: 1-2

Ingredients:

- ¼ cup of coconut or almond cream
- 1 tsp. of maple syrup
- 2 tbsp. of lemon juice
- ½ tbsp. of vegan mustard
- 1 tsp. of poppy seeds
- 1 pinch of salt
- 1 pinch of ground ginger
- 1 tbsp. of spiralized fennel
- ½ cup of spiralized celery
- ½ cup of red grapes without pips cut in two
- 1 red spiralized apple

Preparation:

1. In a big bowl, mix the cream, maple syrup, lemon juice, vegan mustard and poppy seeds until smooth.
2. Add the fennel, celery, grapes and the apple and mix well until the ingredients are well combined.

Dinner Recipes

Vegan Tomato Pasta

<u>Serves: 1-2</u>

<u>Ingredients:</u>

- ¼ teaspoon sea salt
- 1 cup cherry tomatoes
- 1 tablespoon tomato puree
- 1 garlic clove
- 1 tablespoon olive oil
- Spiralized cucumber for garnishing

<u>Preparation:</u>

1. Spiralize the zucchini. Season with salt and massage lightly. Place to one side for the time being.

<u>For the dressing:</u>

1. Mix all the remaining ingredients in a blender and mix until smooth.
2. Add on the sauce and coat evenly.
3. Serve with spiralized cucumber.

Aubergine Pasta with a Creamy Herb Sauce

<u>Serves: 2</u>

<u>Ingredients:</u>

- 3 cups vegan wholegrain noodles

<u>For the sauce:</u>

- 2 aubergines (=eggplants), skin on, sliced
- 1 tbsp. extra virgin olive oil
- 3 tbsp. fresh lemon juice
- ¼ cup organic soy or almond or coconut cream cream
- 1 small garlic clove, grated
- Handful of parsley, chopped
- Handful of pine nuts

<u>Preparation:</u>

1. In a pan cook the sauce in the order listed above until smooth and creamy.
2. Boil the noodles.
3. Pour the sauce over the noodles and mix well to coat.
4. Top with parsley and pine nuts.

Creamy Thai Carrot Noodles

<u>Serves: 1-2</u>

<u>Ingredients:</u>

- 2 large carrots, spiralized into noodles

<u>For the sauce:</u>

- ½ cup coconut milk
- 1 inch piece of ginger
- 1 clove of garlic
- 1 tbsp. masala paste
- 1 tbsp. sesame oil
- Juice and zest of ½ lime
- 1 tsp maple syrup

<u>Preparation:</u>

1. Add all the ingredients for the sauce in the blender and whiz them up until you get a creamy smooth sauce.
2. Spiralize your carrots. You can do this by using a peeler or noodle maker.
3. Toss the carrot noodles in the sauce and serve right away.

Spiralized Mediterranean Couscous

<u>Serves: 2</u>

<u>Ingredients:</u>

- 2 cups of wholegrain couscous
- ¼ cup black olives
- 4 spiralized carrots
- 4 spiralized turnips
- 2 cloves garlic
- ½ cup extra virgin olive oil
- 2 tsp mustard seeds
- 1 tsp balsamic vinegar

<u>Preparation:</u>

1. Peel, wash and spiralize all the vegetables. Mince the garlic. In a saucepan melt the onion and garlic in olive oil.
2. Cook gently for 10 minutes under cover. Add 1 liter of water in the pot, as well as the carrots and turnips. Season.
3. Continue cooking for 15 minutes under cover.
4. Cook the couscous and set aside.
5. Take the veggies off the stove and set to one side for the time being.

6. To serve: Make a couscous dome in a shallow dish on a bed of raisins and some vegetables around. Present in a separate dish the remaining vegetables and their juices in a small bowl.

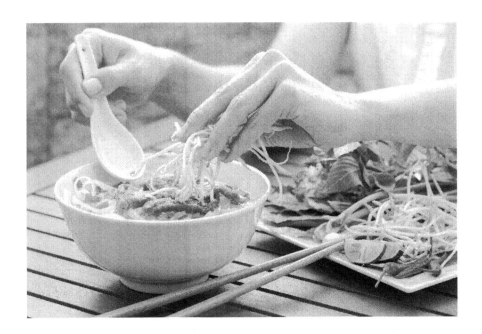

Raw Spiralized Pasta with a Tahini and Tomato Dressing

<u>Serves: 1-2</u>

<u>Ingredients:</u>

- 1 large zucchini
- ¼ teaspoon sea salt
- 5 plum tomatoes
- 3 tbsp. sesame paste
- 1 tbsp. soy shoyu sauce
- 1 tbsp. yeast flakes
- 1 clove of garlic
- 1 tbsp. raw ACV
- 1 tbsp. extra virgin olive oil
- Spiralized cucumber for garnishing

<u>Preparation:</u>

1. Spiralize the zucchini.
2. Season with salt and massage lightly.
3. Set aside while you prepare the dressing.

<u>For the dressing:</u>

1. Mix all remaining ingredients in a blender and combine until smooth.
2. Pour your fresh dressing into the pasta bowl.

3. Now, simply fold the zucchini strands covering each one with the sauce.
4. Dish it up with spiralized cucumber, sliced red pepper or germinated alfalfa.

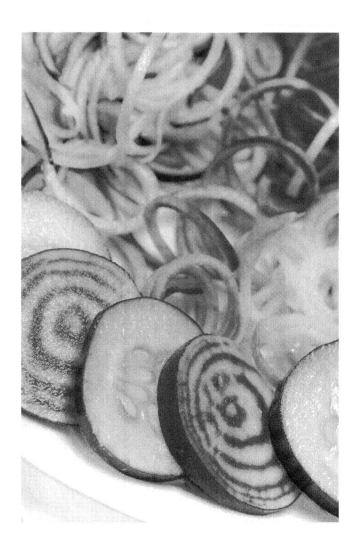

Creamy Garlic Sauce on a Carrot Pasta

<u>Serves:</u>2

<u>Ingredients:</u>

<u>For the noodles:</u>

2 carrots, put through a veggie noodle maker

<u>For the sauce:</u>

- 1 heaped tbsp. of tahini
- 2 tbsps. sweet almond oil
- 3 tbsp. fresh lemon juice
- 1 tsp miso paste
- 1 tsp ground ginger
- 2 garlic cloves, sliced
- Handful of spinach leaves, chopped

<u>Preparation:</u>

1. Cook all of the sauce ingredients until thick.
2. Turn your carrots into noodles using a noodle maker.
3. Add the sauce on the carrot noodles and coat evenly.
4. Garnish with spinach.
5. Serve immediately while hot.

Purple Carrot Noodles with a Thai Sauce

<u>Serves:</u>2

<u>Ingredients:</u>

- 2 big carrots (purple or regular), spiralized into the noodles

<u>For the sauce:</u>

- ½ cup coconut milk (preferably homemade)
- 2cm (3/4 inch) piece of ginger
- 1 clove of garlic
- 1 tbsp. tamari
- 1 tbsp. sesame oil
- Chili, to taste
- Juice and zest of ½ lime
- 1 tsp sweetener (like maple syrup)
- To serve: sesame seeds and fresh mint

<u>Preparation:</u>

1. Blend all of the sauce ingredients until they resemble a smooth consistency.
2. Spiralize your carrots. For this you can use a regular peeler or a noodle maker.

3. Combine the carrot noodles with the sauce until evenly coated.

Linguine of Zucchinis in a Pumpkin and Pistachio Sauce

<u>Serves: 2</u>

<u>Ingredients:</u>

- 3-4 cups of spiralized zucchinis
- 2 cups of cooked pumpkin, puréed
- 1 clove of garlic
- 2 handfuls of whole or powder pistachio nuts
- 2 cans of cream / milk of coconut
- Habanero, hot pepper or other hot pepper of your choice
- Coconut oil
- Pinch of turmeric
- Pinch of salt
- Soy sauce

<u>Preparation:</u>

1. Quickly blanch spiralized zucchinis (linguine thickness) in boiling and slightly salted water during one minute or until wished consistency. Normally, they should remain "al dente".

2. Warm the oil in a big saucepan, add the turmeric. Melt in the oil and add the garlic, for one more minute.

3. Add the cooked pumpkin in the pan, with the coconut cream, the hot pepper and the soy sauce, add a little water if the texture is too dense.

4. Remove of the fire and incorporate the hot pepper into the taste. Add pistachio nuts, well mix.

5. Season with the soy sauce and the salt to the taste. Add directly on the spirals of blanched zucchinis.

Couscous with Spiralized Vegetables

<u>Serves:</u>2

<u>Ingredients:</u>

- 2 cups of medium grain couscous
- 1 small can of chickpeas
- 4 spiralized carrots
- 4 spiralized turnips
- 2 zucchini spiralized
- 2 spiralized onions
- 1 big fennel spiralized
- 1 green pepper and 1 red pepper cut in 4 pieces
- 2 cloves garlic
- 2 tablespoons olive oil
- ½ cup sesame butter and 2 tablespoons of extra virgin olive oil
- 2 tsp of turmeric
- 2 teaspoons coriander seeds
- ¼ cup raisins
- Pinch of salt
- Your favorite vegan-friendly chili sauce

<u>Preparation:</u>

1. Peel, wash and spiralize all vegetables except the peppers (to be cut in 4 big chunks). Spiralize onion and mince the

garlic. In a saucepan melt the onion and garlic in olive oil.

2. Cook gently for 10 minutes under cover. Add 1 liter of water in the pot, as well as chickpeas, carrots and turnips. Salt and pepper.

3. Continue cooking for 15 minutes under cover. Add zucchini, chickpeas, fennel, coriander and turmeric. Continue cooking for 15 minutes under cover.

4. For the couscous it is better to use a couscous maker and steam it then roll it (while warm) in the sesame butter and oil separating the grains but you can use this method as an alternative: Melt the sesame butter and olive oil in a pan, add the couscous. Stir.

5. Take off the heat and add the same amount of water (2 glasses). Let the couscous absorb it then use a fork to separate the grains.

6. To serve: Make a couscous dome in a shallow dish on a bed of raisins and some vegetables around. Present in a separate dish the remaining vegetables and their juices in a small bowl.

Wholegrain Zucchini Spaghetti with Hazelnuts and Kale

Serves: 2

Ingredients:

- 4 oz. spaghetti
- 2 zucchinis
- 4 tablespoons soy or almond butter
- ½ cup hazelnuts, chopped
- 2 cups roughly chopped kale
- 1 tsp salt
- ½ cup vegan cheese
- Salt and pepper to taste

Preparation:

1. Bring a large pot of salted water to a rolling boil. Boil until just cooked. Reserve ½ cup or so of cooking liquid.
2. Turn the zucchini into noodles using a spiralizer attached with a spaghetti blade.
3. In a large skillet, melt soy butter over a medium-high heat. Toast the hazelnuts. Then, add the kale, zucchini and seasoning.
4. Once the kale and zucchini has softened, add spaghetti and vegan cheese. Toss until combined. If necessary, add

a little bit of the cooking liquid to the pan to loosen the sauce up.

5. Season the dish and top with more spiralized carrots.

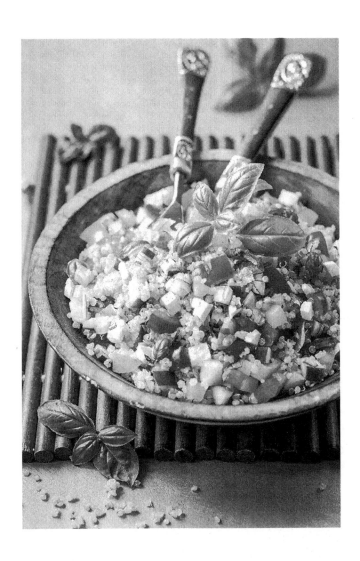

Vegan Coconut Curry

<u>Serves:2</u>

<u>Ingredients:</u>

- 3 tbsp. curry paste
- 1 can of coconut milk
- 2 spiralized broccoli
- 2 spiralized carrots
- 1 spiralized onion
- 1 garlic head chopped
- ½ can chickpeas, drained
- 1 tsp of sesame oil

<u>Preparation:</u>

1. Sauté broccoli, carrots and onion/garlic in a tablespoon of oil. Add the coconut milk after a couple of minutes and let it slightly simmer for a few minutes. The broccoli should be soft yet crispy at the same time.
2. Add the curry paste to the pan and whisk it until it combines with the coconut milk. Add the chickpeas.
3. Add the cornstarch and bring to a boil for about a minute, then reduce the heat to allow the sauce to thicken.

Sweet Potato and Zucchini Pasta with Almonds

<u>Serves:</u>2

<u>Ingredients:</u>

- 1 large sweet potato peeled and spiralized
- 1 zucchini spiralized
- 2 tbsp coconut oil
- 1 tbsp. maple syrup
- Sea salt to taste
- 1 tsp garlic powder or ginger powder or both (optional)
- 1 cup sliced almonds (or chopped pistachios)

<u>Preparation:</u>

1. Peel and spiralize the sweet potato and the zucchini. Then, set aside.
2. Add the zucchini to a large sauté pan with the oil and maple syrup.
3. On a medium to low heat, cook while still covered. Stir every few minutes and add more water to replace the oil and lost water content.
4. They should be soft in about 3 minutes or so. Then add in the sweet potato and sea salt.
5. When the vegetables feel soft take it off the heat and drain.

6. Lastly, add the almonds (or pistachios).

7. Serve hot.

8. Add chili to the taste.

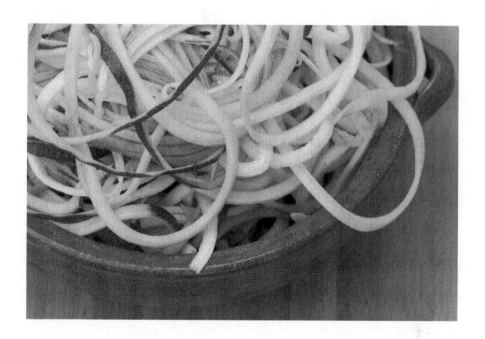

Thai Zucchini and Cucumber Noodle Collard Green Wraps with an Almond Butter Sauce

<u>Serves:2</u>

<u>Ingredients:</u>

<u>For the wraps:</u>

- 5 large collard green leaves, stems removed
- 1 large zucchini, noodles trimmed
- 1 medium cucumber, noodles trimmed
- ¼ cup cilantro leaves
- 1 large bell pepper, sliced thinly
- ½ cup shredded red cabbage

<u>For the almond sauce:</u>

- 1 tsp shredded ginger
- 1 garlic clove, mashed to a paste
- ½ cup creamy almond butter (make sure it's vegan friendly)
- 2 tbsp fresh lime juice
- 2 tbsp. soy sauce, low-sodium
- 1 tsp maple syrup
- 2 tbsp. water

Preparation:

1. Blend all of the ingredients for the sauce until it resembles a smooth and creamy consistency. Then, set aside.

2. On a chopping board, spread out the collard leaf and add a heaped spoon of the sauce, leaving a centimeter of room on the ends for rolling.

3. Add on top the cucumber, cabbage, cilantro and pepper. Carefully roll as you would a wrap and secure the ends with toothpicks.

4. Repeat for the rest of the leaves and slice in half before serving up. Add the remaining sauce to your plate as a dip.

Snacks and Treats

Grilled Eggplant Stacks on Kale and Spiralized Sweet Potato Chips

Serves:2-4

Kale and sweet potato chips:

Ingredients:

- 6 cups torn stemmed kale

- 2 cups of spiralized sweet potatoes

- 3 tsp olive oil

- 1 pinch salt

- 1 pinch sweet curry powder or a blend of turmeric, paprika, cloves, cardamom and cumin

Preparation:

1. Toss together kale, spiralized sweet potatoes, oil, salt and paprika

2. Arrange in single layer on parchment paper–lined baking sheet.

3. Bake in 350F (180C) oven until the kale is crisp and dark green and the sweet potatoes softly crispy, for 12-15 minutes.

Grilled eggplants stacks:

Get the most out of eggplant by grilling it to bring out the most flavor.

- 2x1 pound of eggplants (you will need to slice them into 12 rounds each, 1/3- to 1/2-inch thick)
- Coarse salt, such as kosher or sea salt, for sprinkling
- 1/2 cup olive oil
- 1 can of tomato sauce
- Parsley (minced)

Preparation:

1. In a colander place the eggplants evenly and apply sea salt. Leave the colander in the sink you drain out any leftover juices and dry with a clean cloth.
2. In the meantime, heat the grill to a medium setting.
3. Spray the oil over the eggplants and grill for 10 minutes or until soft. Turn every minutes for an even consistency. Add more salt while doing this.
4. The best way to serve is: stack 4 eggplant slices (per one serving) with a drizzle of tomato sauce (make it generous) sandwiched between each layer.
5. What we want is that some sauce is visible between layers.
6. Add an even dollop of sauce to each eggplant and garnish before serving.

7. Serve while still hot on a bed of kale and sweet potatoes chips.

Remember to get your free, complimentary smoothie recipe PDF eBook (100% vegan):

www.holisticwellnessbooks.com/vegan

Spiralized Mango Salad

Serves:1-2

Ingredients:

- 1 mango, cut in half and spiralized
- 1 pear spiralized
- Organic dairy-free yoghurt
- 1 tbsp. desiccated coconut

Preparation:

1. Mix all of the ingredients, except the mango and let it sit for 30 minutes.
2. Serve in champagne glasses and top it with a dash of maple syrup.

Pear Crisps

Serves: 2

Ingredients:

•2 tbsp. of almond butter, melted

•3 tbsp. coconut milk

•¼ tsp cinnamon

•1-2 tbsp. chopped walnuts

•2 tbsp. desiccated coconut

•Drizzle of agave syrup

•1 pear

Preparation:

For the sauce:

1. Take a small-medium bowl and mix together the almond butter and the coconut milk until smooth.

2. Stir in the cinnamon. Set aside.

3. Heat a small skillet (medium heat).

4. Add walnuts.

5. Now toast for a few minutes, until nicely browned and fragrant.

6. Take off from the heat and let it cool.

7. Add the desiccated coconut to the skillet and toast briefly.

8. Take off from the stove and set one side.

9. Slice your pear using the largest blade on the spiralizer. (half

the pear)

10. Now, drizzle the slices with lemon juice to prevent browning. Repeat the process with the other half.

11. Spread the pear slices out on a large plate. Drizzle the almond sauce over top, then sprinkle on the walnuts. Finish with a tiny drizzle of agave syrup if desired.

Turnip and Carrot Pasta with Almonds

<u>Serves: 1-2</u>

<u>Ingredients:</u>

- 1 large turnip peeled and spiralized
- 1 carrot spiralized
- 2 tbsp. coconut oil
- 1 tbsp. maple syrup
- Sea salt to taste
- 1 tsp garlic powder or ginger powder or both (optional)
- 1 cup sliced almonds (or chopped pistachios)

<u>Preparation:</u>

1. Peel the sweet potato and spiralize it. Spiralize the zucchini. Set aside.
2. Add the zucchini to a large sauté pan with the oil and maple syrup.
3. Cook covered on medium to low heat. You may need to add a little extra oil or some water if the oil cooks off. Keep a close eye on them and stir every couple minutes.
4. They should be soft in about 3 minutes or so. Then add in the sweet potato and sea salt.
5. Stir together for another couple minutes until everything looks softened. Lastly, add the almonds (or pistachios). Serve immediately or refrigerate for later.
6. Add chili to the taste.

Kidney Bean, Sweet Potato Sweet & Spicy Wrap

<u>Serves:2</u>

<u>Ingredients:</u>

<u>For the wraps:</u>

- 5 large collard green leaves, stems removed
- 1 clove garlic, minced
- 1 (15-ounce) can black beans
- 1 tablespoon olive oil
- ¼ teaspoon smoked paprika
- ½ cup shredded red cabbage

<u>For the sweet potato:</u>

- 1 large sweet potato (about 1 pound), peeled and sliced into 1/4-inch thick rounds
- 1 garlic clove, mashed to a paste
- 1 tablespoon olive oil
- Salt and pepper to taste
- 1 teaspoon ground cumin

<u>Preparation:</u>

1. In a blender, combine all of the ingredients for the sweet potato and set aside.

2. Fold out flat, the collard leaves and add a tablespoon of olive oil on each one.

3. On top, add the sweet potato, cumin, cilantro, garlic, cabbage, black beans and paprika.

4. Delicately fold the leaves like you would with a burrito and hold in place with toothpicks.

5. Repeat with remaining collard green leaves and then slice both in half and serve.

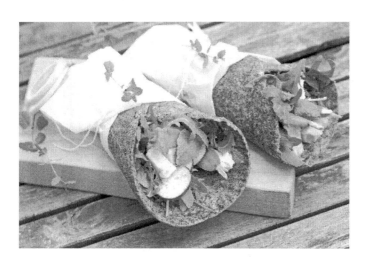

Apple Nachos

Ingredients:

•2 tbsp. of cashew butter, melted

•3 tbsp. coconut milk

•¼ tsp nutmeg

•¼ cup walnuts, chopped

•1 tbsp. desiccated coconut

•1 apple, cored

•2 tbsp. agave syrup

•Lemon juice

Preparation:

Begin with the sauce:

1. In a small bowl, whisk or stir together the cashew butter and the coconut milk until smooth.

2. Stir in the nutmeg and set aside for now.

3. Heat a small skillet on the stove over medium heat.

4. Add the walnuts and toast for a few minutes, until browned and fragrant. Remove from pan and cool.

5. Add the desiccated coconut to the skillet and toast briefly, just as soon as they start to turn down.

6. Take off the heat and for the time-being set to one side.

7. Using the largest blade on your spiralizer, carve the apples.

8. Once you've gone through half of the apple, drizzle the slices with lemon juice to prevent browning. Once you're done carving the apple, drizzle the rest of the lemon on your slices to prevent them from browning.

9. Spread the apple slices out on a large plate. Pour the sauce on top and add on the desiccated coconut and walnuts.

Spring Rolls

Here is a delicious way to use leafy vegetables which are quite seasonal. With a little imagination, collard, kale or chard leaves are transformed into delicious "wraps", burritos, sandwiches, spring rolls ... it takes only a little practice to get to do rolls like pros!

To imitate the spring rolls you usually do in a rice paper, stuff cabbage leaves of collard with daikon radish noodles (made with spiralizer) and a blend of:

Serves:2
Ingredients:

- Mango, julienned
- Cucumber, julienned
- Marinated mushrooms (in tamari and sesame oil)
- Spiralized carrots
- Coriander leaves (or mint or basil)
- Avocado slices

And serve with a choice of sauces:
tahini sauce with white miso:

- 2 teaspoons of white miso
- 2 tablespoons lemon juice tea

- 1 teaspoon of tahini
- 1-2 tablespoons of water table
- Garlic and ginger

Mix all ingredients gently with a fork.

Almond sauce:
- 1 tablespoon almond butter
- 1 tablespoon water
- 1 tablespoon lemon juice
- 1 teaspoon tamari
- 1 teaspoon of maple syrup

Preparation:
1. Stir with a fork, add a little more water if the sauce is too thick.
2. Place all ingredients in electric mini-chopper or food processor until a smooth sauce. Season to your taste.

Vegan Eggplant Caviar Dip

<u>Serves:</u>2

<u>Ingredients:</u>

- 2 medium eggplants
- 1 large clove garlic, minced to a paste
- 1 ¼ teaspoons
- Pinch of salt
- 2 tablespoons tahini
- 3 tablespoons of olive oil
- Juice of 1 lemon

<u>Preparation:</u>

1. Heat the oven to 375°F.
2. Place the eggplants on a foil-lined baking sheet. Broil for 25-30 min until the skin is slightly burned, wrinkled or until the eggplants are very tender.
3. Let the eggplants cool for about 15 minutes, until cool enough to handle. Slit them open and scoop out the flesh, leaving all the skin behind. Transfer the flesh to a bowl. Break down into a purée.
4. Add the minced garlic, tahini, 2 tablespoons olive oil and the juice of 1 lemon. Stir to distribute, you'll see the dip get creamy as you stir. Taste to balance the flavors, adding more olive oil, lemon juice, or salt to taste. Serve

as is, let it cool to room temperature or store in the fridge and eat cold.

5. Serve as a dip with spiralized veggies of your choice.

Remember to get your free, complimentary smoothie recipe PDF eBook (100% vegan):

www.holisticwellnessbooks.com/vegan

Wholegrain Seeded Rice with Spiralized Avocado

<u>Serves:</u>2

<u>Ingredients:</u>

- 1 avocado, cut in half and spiralized
- 1 ½ cups brown rice
- 1 cup of mixed seeds
- 1 tbsp. balsamic vinegar

<u>Preparation:</u>

1. Spiralize the avocado.
2. Boil the rice until soft and strain.
3. In a salad bowl add the cooked rice and add the mixed seeds on top.
4. Then drizzle on the balsamic vinegar. Garnish with spiralized avocado.

Quick Moroccan Spiralized Carrot Dish

<u>Serves:2</u>

<u>Ingredients:</u>

- 5 large carrots, peeled
- 1 tbsp. extra virgin olive oil   or coconut oil
- 1 tbsp. garlic powder
- 2 tsp nutmeg
- 2 tsp ground turmeric
- 1 tbsp. grated ginger
- 3 tbsp ground coriander
- Pinch of salt & pepper

<u>Preparation:</u>

1. Using your spiralizer carve out your carrots into long slices.
2. In a frying pan cook your olive oil, carrots, garlic powder and cook for a few minutes on a medium to low heat.
3. Add the salt and pepper and cook for further 5 minutes.
4. Sprinkle the remaining ingredients on top and serve on hot plates.

Root Vegetable Chips

<u>Serves:2</u>

<u>Ingredients:</u>

- 1 parsnip
- 1 sweet potatoes
- beets
- 1 celeriac
- 1 tbsp. olive oil
- Pinch of salt to taste

<u>Preparation:</u>

1. Heat the oven to 375F.(190 Celsius)
2. Peel and spiralize all vegetables with the blade to slice.
3. Put and tap on a paper towel and add salt. Let stand for 15 minutes.
4. Cover two baking sheets with parchment paper.
5. Put the vegetable slices in a single floor.
6. Spray with oil or use a brush
7. Add salt
8. Bake for 20 min. Depending on the thickness of the cooking time may vary. Keep an eye on your chips and remove them as they seem and smell cooked.
9. Repeat.

Scalloped Potatoes

<u>Serves: 2</u>

<u>Ingredients:</u>

- Olive oil cooking spray
- 1 garlic clove
- 1 tbsp. organic Earth Balance
- ¼ lbs. golden potatoes
- 1 small onion, sliced
- cups non-dairy creamer
- ¾ tbsp. salt
- Freshly ground pepper
- 1 cup of vegan soy cheese, shredded

<u>Preparation:</u>

1. Ready the oven to 375F.
2. Grease a casserole dish with garlic. Set aside for a few minutes to dry. Spray the olive oil (or other cooking spray) around the inside of the dish.
3. Peel and slice the potatoes with a peeler. In a large saucepan combine the Erath balance, seasoning, non dairy creamer and remaining garlic. Simmer for 5 minutes and place into the pre-greased dish. Sprinkle with cheese and bake until golden and crisp.
4. Cool slightly before serving.

Crispy Curled Fries

Serves: 2

Ingredients:

- large white potatoes, washed & dried
- 1 tbsp. extra virgin olive oil
- 1 tsp sea salt

Preparation:

1. Heat the oven to 375F. (190 Celsius)
2. Carve the potatoes using the triangular blade on the spiralizer.
3. Cover the potato slices with olive oil
4. Apply over 2 sheets of baking paper.
5. Season with sea salt.
6. Bake for 10-15 minutes.
7. Remove from the oven once crisp and serve hot.

Note: If you would like to add fresh herbs, sprinkle them over fries in between baking, before you place them back in the oven for 8-10 minutes. Use Jerusalem artichoke. As it cooks more quickly, reduce baking time to 6-7 minutes.

Steamed Jerusalem Artichoke

<u>Serves:</u>2

<u>Ingredients:</u>

- 2 cups of spiralized Jerusalem artichokes
- Salt or soy sauce
- 1 tbsp. of almond butter

<u>Preparation:</u>

1. Steam the spiralized Jerusalem artichoke for 5 to 6 minutes Add seasoning and almond butter.
2. Sprinkle with chopped parsley or cilantro.
3. Enjoy!

Roasted Spiralized Root Veggies

<u>Serves:2-4</u>

<u>Ingredients:</u>

- 1 medium celeriac
- 6 parsnips small or medium, peeled, cut lengthwise into 2
- 6 carrots, peeled, cut into 2 lengthwise
- 3 tbsp. extra virgin olive oil
- 1 head garlic, cloves in defeat, peeled
- sprigs of rosemary, leaves only
- To taste sea salt and freshly ground pepper
- To taste, cilantro, basil or parsley, chopped

<u>Preparation:</u>

1. Preheat oven to 350 ° F. (175 Celsius)
2. Meanwhile, put the celeriac under cold water and peel. Cut into pieces and blanch for 5 minutes. Drain and set aside.
3. In a shallow baking dish, pour the oil to coat the bottom. Add the garlic, rosemary leaves and season with sea salt and pepper. Add in the vegetables and coat well by stirring in the seasoned oil. Vegetables should be placed in a single layer and not stacked so that they are well roasted. Pour a little olive oil over the vegetables.

4. Increase the temperature to 400 °F and cook the vegetables for 15 minutes. Vegetables should be tender and golden. Sprinkle with chopped fresh herbs just before serving.

Remember to get your free, complimentary smoothie recipe PDF eBook (100% vegan):

www.holisticwellnessbooks.com/vegan

Marinated Spiralized Beets

<u>Serves:</u> 2

<u>Ingredients:</u>

- 4 lbs. of beets
- cups raw cider vinegar
- 1 ½ cup of agave syrup
- 1 tbsp. of mustard seeds
- 1 tsp. of sea salt

<u>Preparation:</u>

1. Peel the beets and spiralize them in large rolls. Take a large pan and cook the beets' spirals, until they are tender, about 20-30 min. Reserve 1 cup (250 ml) of filtered cooking water. Dive beets spirals in cold water. Reserve.

2. In another saucepan, bring the reserved cooking water, vinegar, sugar, mustard seeds and salt.

3. Put the beets into sterilized jars and cover with boiling marinade. Seal well. Sterilize if desired (Put jars 35 minutes in boiling water).

Cashew Rice with a Coconut Dressing

<u>Serves:</u> 2

<u>Ingredients:</u>

- 1 tbsp. cashew butter
- 2/3 cup onion, chopped
- 1 ½ cups cooked brown rice
- 1 tsp curry powder
- cups coconut milk
- 1 cup vegan veggie broth
- ¼ cup cashews, toasted
- Finely spiralized veggies (for example: carrots and bok choy or similar)

<u>Preparation:</u>

1. Melt the butter in a saucepan. Cook the onion until it's golden brown and soft. Add the curry powder and rice. Cook for a further minute.
2. Add coconut milk and veggie broth and boil uncovered about 5 minutes.
3. When you see air holes forming, add the thinly spiralized veggies. Cover immediately, reduce to a low heat and simmer for 10 minutes with the lid covered.
4. Let it sit for 10 minutes, then mix in the cashews.

Spiralized Dragon Fruit Salad

Dragon fruit can be spiralized!

As an alkaline food, it can be enjoyed in fruit salads or in combination with slightly less alkaline yet healthy foods as it is recommended that you consume 70-80% alkaline foods to optimize and energize your body and avoid health problems.

Pears and apples are two other fruits that are easily spiralized. Use the three fruits in a delicious and colorful fruit salad.

Serves: 2

Ingredients:

- 1 dragon fruit (not completely ripe) spiralized in noodle
- 1 apple, spiralized (or sliced with the spiralizer)
- 1 pear spiralized
- 1 honey dew melon (in small balls)
- A cup of pineapple juice
- 6 mint leaves, roughly chopped
- Soy yoghurt, or coconut yoghurt, and/or and maple syrup for topping

Preparation:

1. Blend all of the ingredients except the ones for topping and let it sit for 30 minutes.
2. Serve in champagne glasses and top it with soy yoghurt and a dash of maple syrup.

Marinated Spiralized Cucumber

<u>Serves:2</u>

<u>Ingredients:</u>

- 4 lbs. of cucumber
- 2 cups raw cider vinegar
- 1 tbsp. of mustard seeds
- 1 tsp. of sea salt

<u>Preparation:</u>

1. Spiralize the cucumbers.
2. In a bowl, combine the vinegar, mustard seeds and salt.
3. Put the cucumbers into sterilized jars and pour over the marinade.
4. Seal well. Can keep to up to 2 weeks in the fridge.

BONUS CONTENT: Vegan Gluten-Free Recipes

Toasted Chickpeas

Chickpeas are a great source of protein, healthy carbohydrates and fiber. This recipe provides you with a much more nutritious option to a bag of commercially made potato chips, that we so often find ourselves grabbing when hunger strikes during a trip to the grocery store. These toasted chickpeas can be made in advance and easily stored in a glass jar or handbag/briefcase sized container. Their tasty crunch is bound to satisfy any snack craving. They also make a great crunchy protein-packed addition to your lunchtime salad.

Makes four ¼ Cup servings
Ingredients:

- 1 Can Chickpeas, drained and rinsed

- 1 Teaspoon Ground Organic Sea Salt

- 1 Teaspoon Ground Black Pepper

- 1 Teaspoon Organic dried herb mix

- 1 Tablespoon Extra Virgin Olive oil

Instructions:

1. Drain and rinse the chickpeas in a colander

2. Pour the chickpeas into a mixing bowl and add the sea salt, black pepper and dried herb mix

3. Toss together well

4. Pour the olive oil over a piece of kitchen paper towel and rub it over a non-stick baking sheet

5. Place the chickpeas onto the baking sheet

6. Turn your oven onto to grill

7. Once the grill element is nice and hot, place the baking sheet with the chickpeas on it under the grill

8. Grill for approximately 25-30minutes, the idea is that the chickpeas lose all their moisture and become browned and crunchy.

Baked Falafel Balls

These falafel balls are another protein-packed, tasty snack option that can be served with any of the above hummus variations. They also make a great protein addition to your lunchtime salad. Because these falafel balls are baked as opposed to the usual method of frying, they are a healthier alternative. Make them in advance and store them in the refrigerator, they can also be frozen.

Makes approximately 45 balls
Ingredients:

- 4 Cans Chickpeas, drained and rinsed

- 2 Teaspoons Ground Organic Sea Salt

- 2 Teaspoons Ground Black Pepper

- 2 Teaspoons Baking Powder

- 1 Teaspoon Cumin Seeds

- 1 Teaspoon Fresh Coriander, finely chopped

- 1 Teaspoon Cayenne Pepper

- 1 Tablespoon Fresh Garlic, finely chopped

- 1 Tablespoon Fresh Ginger root, finely chopped

- ¼ Cup Lemon Juice

- ¼ Cup Tahini

- 1 Tablespoon Extra Virgin Coconut Oil

Instructions:

1. Preheat the oven to 350 degrees (200 degrees Celsius)

2. Place all the ingredients into the food processor and blitz until smooth

3. Place the ingredients into a bowl and refrigerate for about ½ hour, until the mixture has firmed up

4. Using a piece of kitchen paper towel, pour the coconut oil over the paper towel and grease a non-stick baking sheet with it

5. Form the falafel mixture into balls, about the size of a large marble and place the balls onto the baking sheet

6. Bake for 30-35 minutes or until golden brown. Ensure that you turn the balls over half way through cooking.

Fresh Fruit Skewers with Vegan Coconut Yoghurt Dip

Fruit is an incredibly healthy and nutritious snack alternative to sugar laden sweets. The natural sugars in fruits are slowly released and therefore help in maintaining blood sugar without giving you that horrible spike that comes from refined sugar. These skewers are easy to prepare in advance and make a great addition to any lunch box or picnic basket. The coconut yoghurt dip not only adds protein, but also a little extra comfort to this snack combination.

Makes approximately 10 Skewers

Ingredients to make the fruit skewers:

- 1 medium sized fresh papaya, peeled, pitted and cubed

- 1 medium sized fresh pineapple, peeled and cubed

- 1 Cup fresh white seedless grapes, whole

- 1 Cup fresh black seedless grapes, whole

- 1 Cup whole dates

Instructions to make the fruit skewers:

1. Using either wooden or bamboo skewer sticks place the fruit pieces on the skewer sticks, alternating with a

single piece of the different fruits at a time. For example, 1 piece papaya, 1 piece pineapple, 1 white grape, 1 date, 1 red grape.

2. Continue until the skewer is full and then begin the next one

3. Once all the fruit is has been skewered, place the fruit skewers on a serving plate or into a tub for refrigeration.

Ingredients to make the vegan yoghurt dip:

- 1 Cup vegan coconut yogurt (or other vegan yoghurt of your choice)

- ¼ Cup Coconut Cream

- 1 Teaspoon Vanilla Essence

- ½ Teaspoon Ground Cinnamon

- 1 Teaspoon Raw Cocoa Powder

- 1 Tablespoon Desiccated Coconut

- 1 Tablespoon Dried Berry mix

Instructions to make the vegan yoghurt dip:

1. Place the yoghurt and coconut cream into a mixing bowl

2. Add the vanilla essence, ground cinnamon and raw cocoa powder

3. Whisk well

4. Stir in the desiccated coconut and the dried berry mix

5. If you are serving the fruit skewers at home then place the yoghurt dip into a serving dish. If you are taking the skewers to go, then place the yoghurt dip into a take away container. Both the yoghurt dip and the fruit skewers are best kept refrigerated, so if you are taking them in your lunch box or to a picnic, ensure that they are in a cooler bag.

Fresh Basil, Cherry Tomato and Herbed Tofu Salad with Pine nuts

There is just something amazing about the flavor combination of tomato and basil. This salad is a tasty, nutritious reason to take a break from your desk.

Serves One:

Ingredients:

- 1 Cup Cooked, diced firm tofu

- ½ Cup Fresh Basil leaves

- ½ Cup Cherry tomatoes, halved

- 1 Tablespoon Raw Pine nuts

- 2 Teaspoons Organic Extra Virgin Olive Oil

Instructions:

1. In a serving bowl, or take away tub, place the fresh basil leaves

2. Add the halved cherry tomatoes

3. Add the cooked tofu

4. Top with the raw pine nuts

5. Just before serving drizzle with the olive oil and toss well. Salt and pepper can be added to taste.

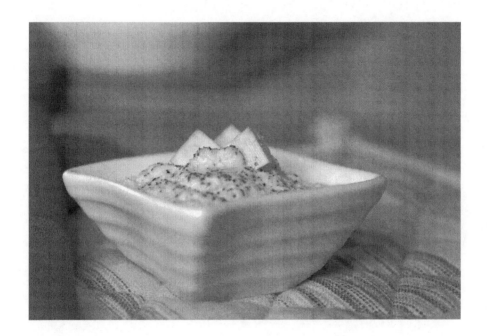

Red Cabbage, Chick Pea and Pomegranate Salad with Pomegranate dressing

Red cabbage not only provides great color to this dish, but it is high in fiber, so will help keep you full all afternoon. Pomegranates are high in antioxidants and are considered a super food.

Serves One:

Ingredients for the salad:

- 1 Cup Raw Red Cabbage, shredded

- ½ Cup Chick peas (can be the canned variety, just make sure you rinse them well)

- ¼ Cup Pomegranate Seeds

- 1 Tablespoon Raw Seed Mix

Ingredients for the dressing:

- ¼ Cup Fresh pomegranate juice

- 1 Tablespoon Extra Virgin Coconut Oil

- ¼ Teaspoon Organic Ground Sea Salt

- ¼ Teaspoon Ground Black Pepper

Instructions to make the salad:

1. In a serving bowl, or a take away tub, place the raw red cabbage

2. Add the chick peas

3. Add the pomegranate seeds

4. Add the raw seed mix

Instructions to make the dressing:

1. In a large mixing jug combine the pomegranate juice, coconut oil, salt and pepper.

2. Whisk well

3. Just before serving, pour the dressing over the salad and toss together

Homemade Trail Mix

Trail mix is another great on-the-go snack option, but very often the pre-packed versions that we buy in the supermarkets contain unnecessary additives and preservatives. By mixing your own trail mix, using organic, raw ingredients you are ensuring that you get a healthy, energy-boosting snack that you can trust. This recipe includes dried berry mix and raw cocoa nibs, making it a great source of anti-oxidants as well.

Makes approximately 4 ¼ Cup
Ingredients:

- 4 Tablespoons   Raw Cashew Nuts, whole

- 4 Tablespoons Raw Brazil Nuts, Whole

- 4 Tablespoons Raw Seed mix

- 4 Tablespoons Dried Berry Mix

- 4 Tablespoons Coconut Flakes

- 4 Tablespoons Raw Cocoa Nibs

- 4 Tablespoons Dried Mango Pieces

- 4 Tablespoons Dried Apple Pieces

Instructions:

1. Place all the ingredients into a large mixing bowl and toss together well

2. Using a ¼ cup measuring cup, divide the trail mix into portions

3. You can either place each portion in a small sandwich bag, or a small take away tub.

4. If you choose not to pre-portion out the entire mix, then you can store it in an airtight glass jar.

Your Free Gift

Don't forget to download your free complimentary recipe eBook:

www.holisticwellnessbooks.com/vegan

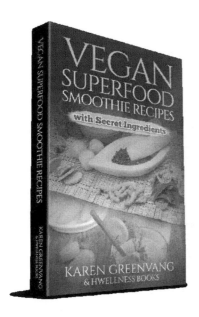

If you have any problems with your download, email me at: karenveganbooks@gmail.com

Conclusion

Thank you for reading!
I hope that with so many vegan recipes you will be
motivated and inspired to start and/or continue
your journey towards meaningful veganism, vibrant
health and total wellbeing.

Remember, the beauty of incorporating nutritious
vegan foods into your daily diet is that you are
making simple, yet sustainable changes that will
work for your wellness long-term. Not to mention
your spiritual wellness and taking care of the
environment.

If you enjoyed my book, it would be greatly
appreciated if you left a review so others can receive
the same benefits you have. Your review can help
other people take this important step to take care of
their health and inspire them to start a new chapter
in their lives.

At the same time, <u>you can help me serve you and all
my other readers</u> even more through my next
vegan-friendly recipe books that I am committed to
publishing on a regular basis.

I'd be thrilled to hear from you. I would love to know your favorite recipe(s).

Don't be shy, post a comment on Amazon! Your comments are really important to me.

→ Questions about this book? Email me at: karenveganbooks@gmail.com

Thank You for your time,

Love & Light,

Until next time-

Karen Vegan Greenvang

www.amazon.com/author/karengreenvang

More Vegan Books by Karen

Available in kindle and paperback in all Amazon stores.

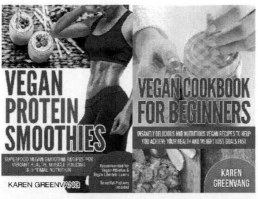

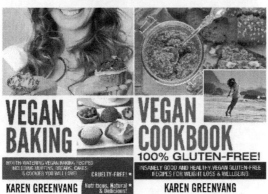

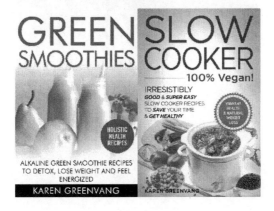

Made in the USA
Middletown, DE
21 December 2017